Miffy's Baby Book

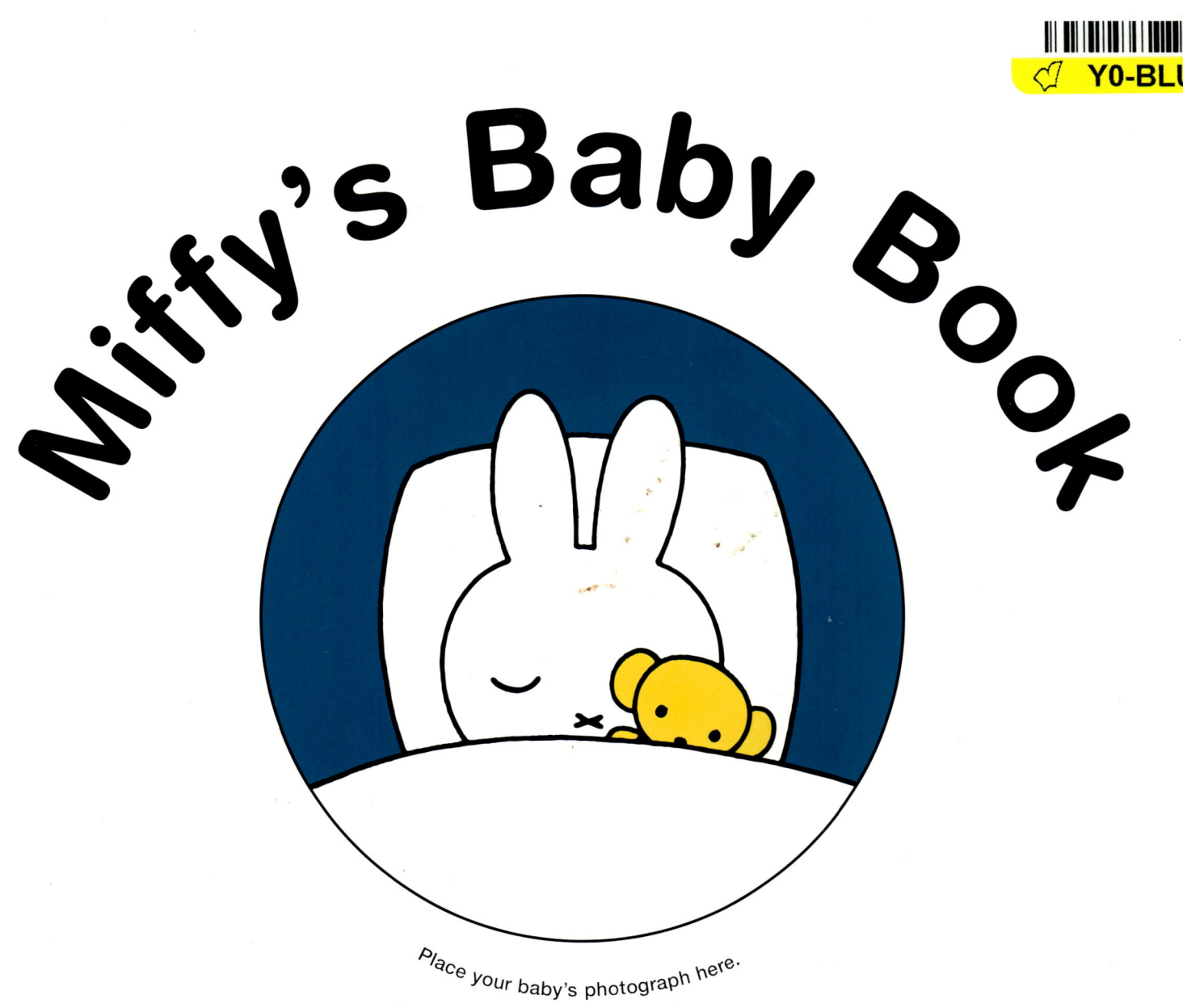

Place your baby's photograph here.

Dick Bruna

Baby's Birth

Baby was born on ....

Time of birth .... am pm

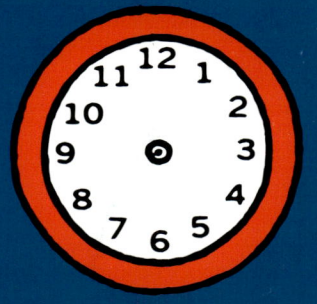

Place of birth ....

Weight at birth ....

Length at birth .... cm

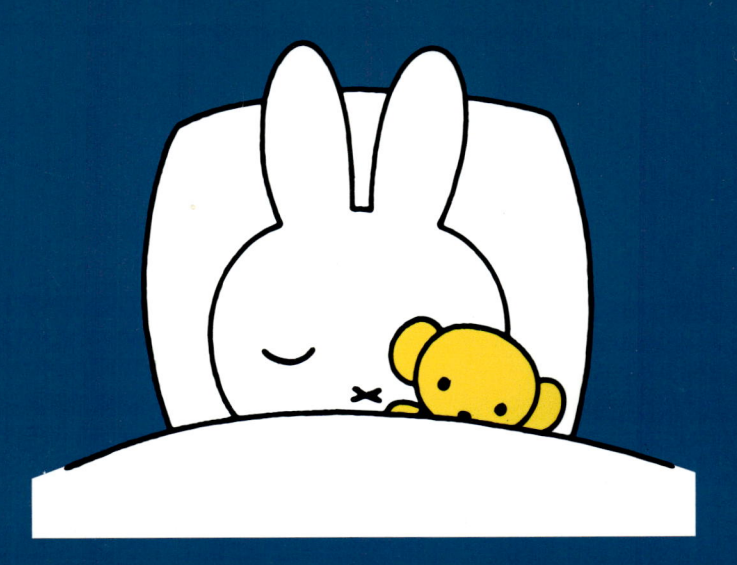

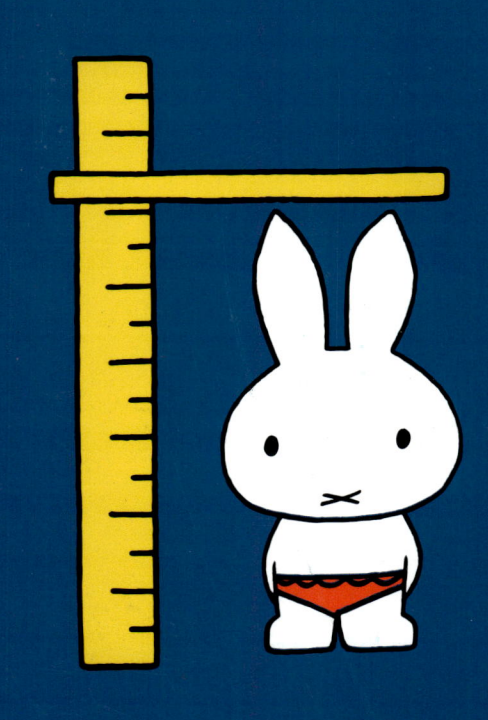

A Beautiful Baby

Photograph

Photograph

Colour of hair
....

Lock of hair

Very first photograph of Baby

Mummy or Daddy as a baby

Baby looks most like ....
....

Welcoming the Baby

Who was present at the birth? ....

First visitors

....

....

Pressed flowers

Cards and gifts from

....

....

....

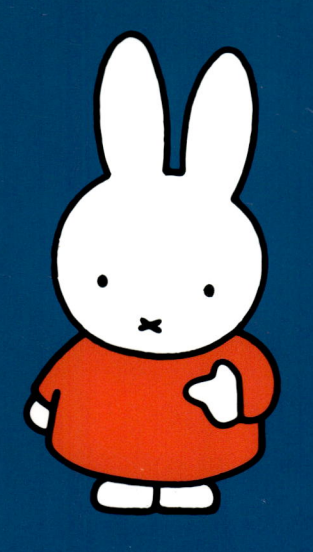

Baby's Name

Baby's name is ....

Chosen because ....

Other names suggested for Baby were

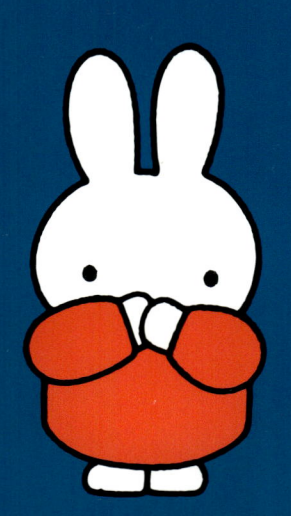

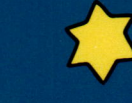

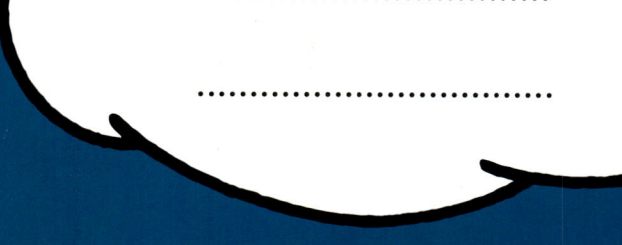

....

....

....

Tiny hands and feet!

Baby's hands are so small they look like this...

and Baby's feet are so tiny they look like this...

Handprint

Footprint

Coming Home

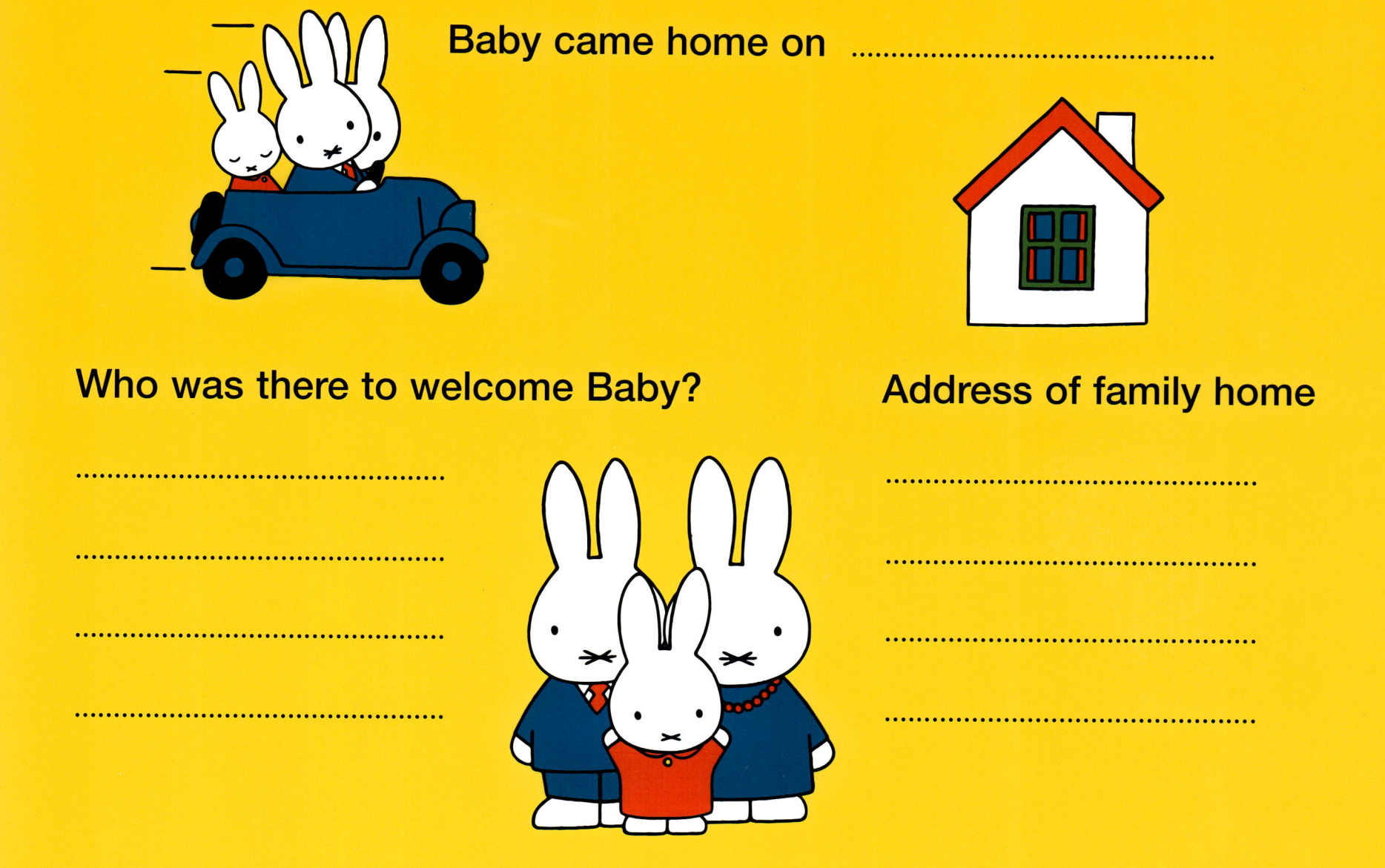

Baby came home on ....

Who was there to welcome Baby?

Address of family home

....

....

....

....

....

....

....

....

Thoughts to Treasure

Mummy thought

....
....
....
....
....

Daddy thought

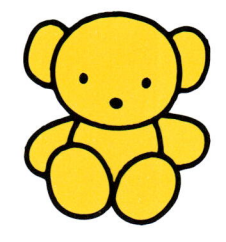

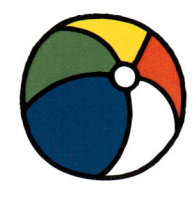

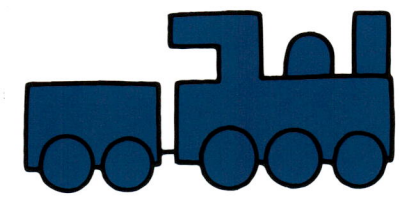

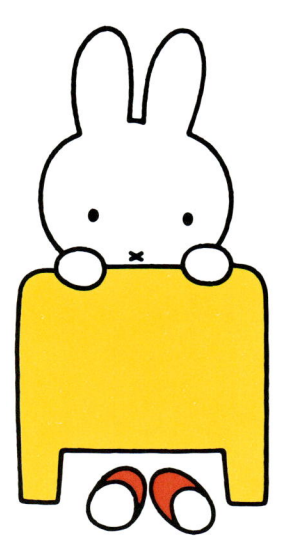

....
....
....
....
....

And Memories to Keep

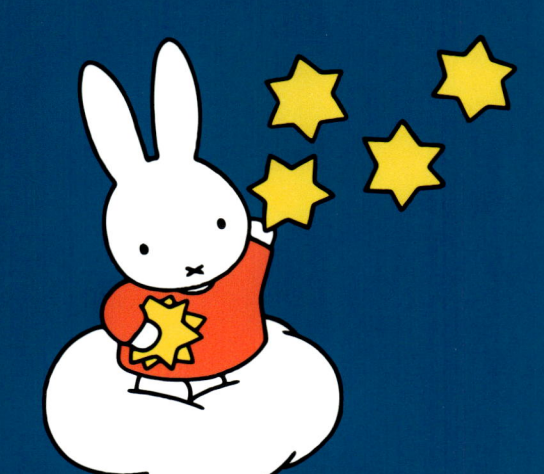

Special memories

....

....

A favourite photograph of Baby

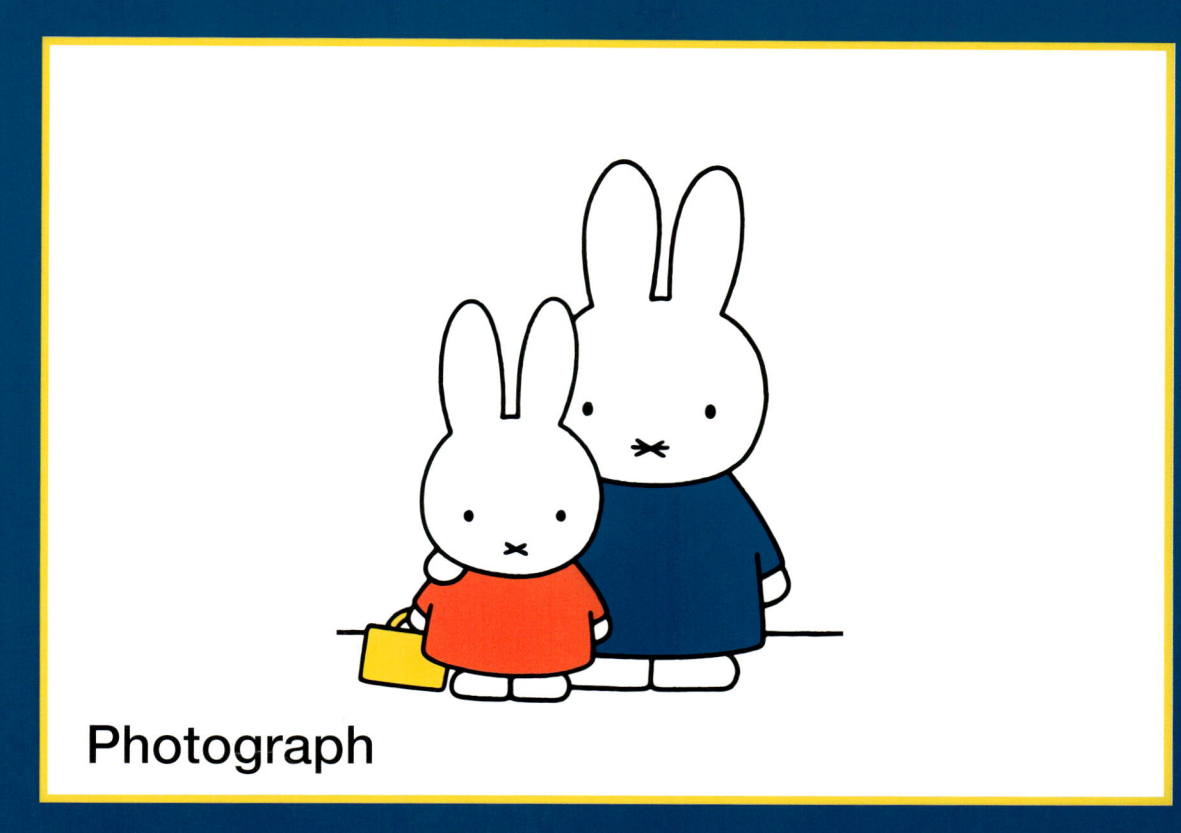

Photograph

Early Days

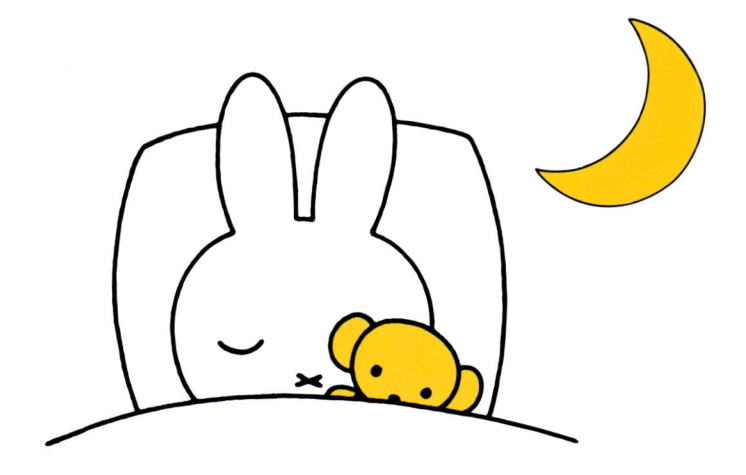

Baby sleeps ....
....

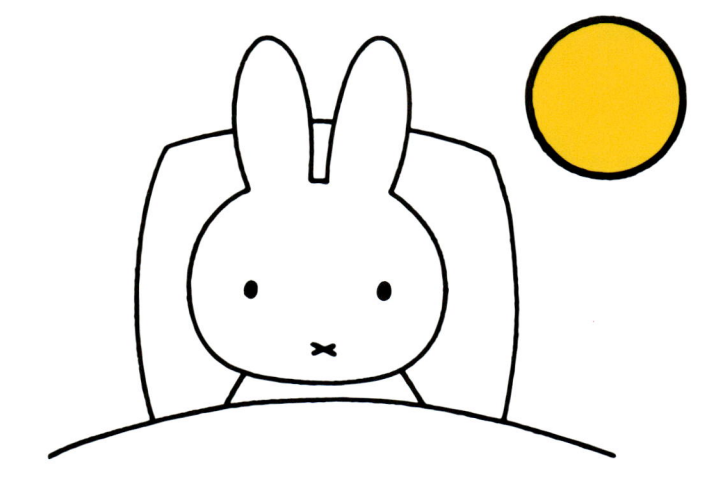

Baby wakes ....
....

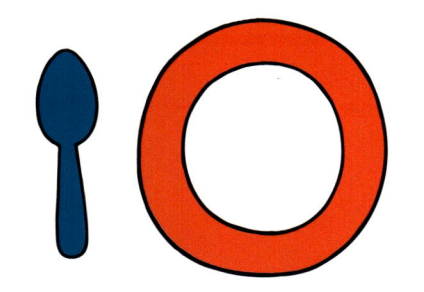

Baby's feeding times ....

....

....

....

The Family

Photograph

Family photograph

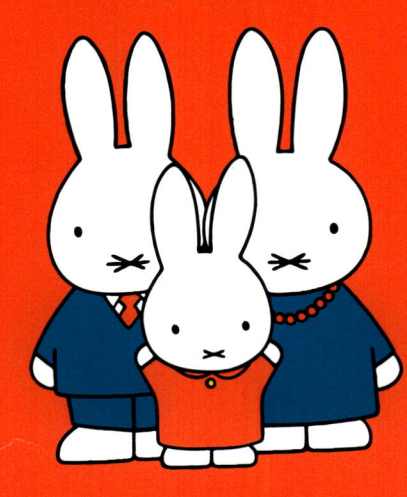

Photograph

Mummy and Daddy

Photograph

Brothers and Sisters

Baby's First Celebration!

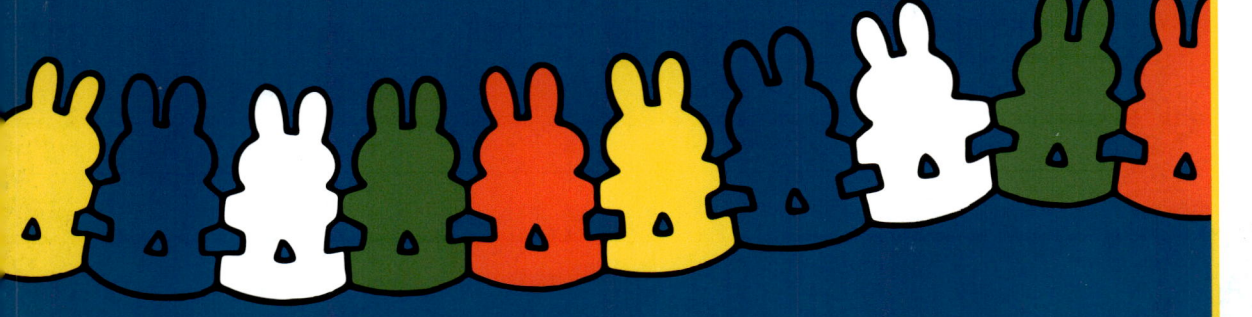

Photograph

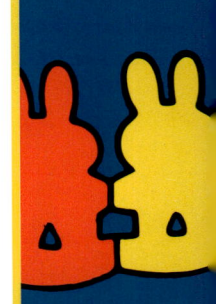

Date of Christening
or Name Day celebration ....

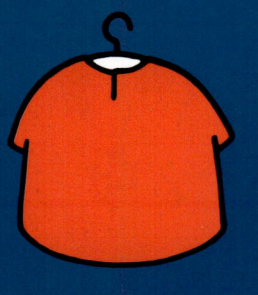

Baby wore ....

....

Gifts received

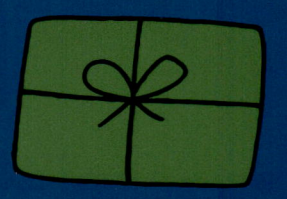

....

....

....

Special guests ....

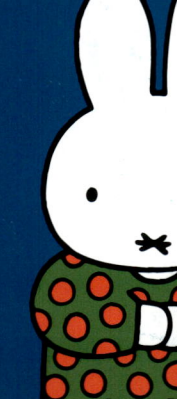

....

....

Baby's Progress

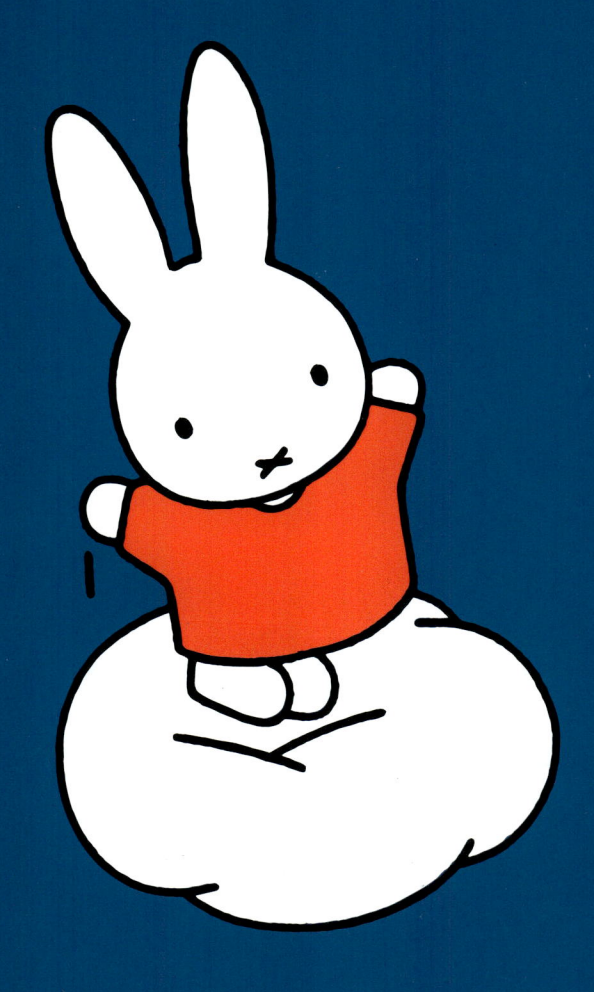

How Baby has changed

....

....

Describe Baby's first weeks

....

....

Favourite activities

....

....

Days out with Baby

Photograph

First trips out are ....

....

....

Bathtime

First bath at home ....

First time in the big bath ....

Favourite bath games ....

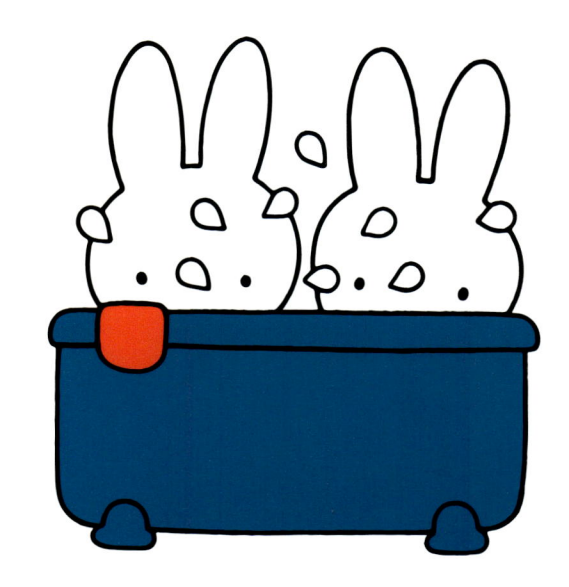

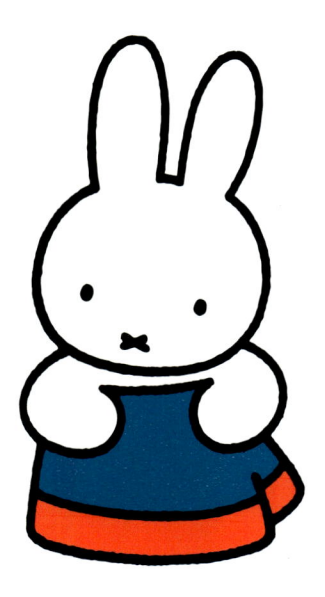

Photograph

Bedtime

Sleeping times ....

First slept through the night

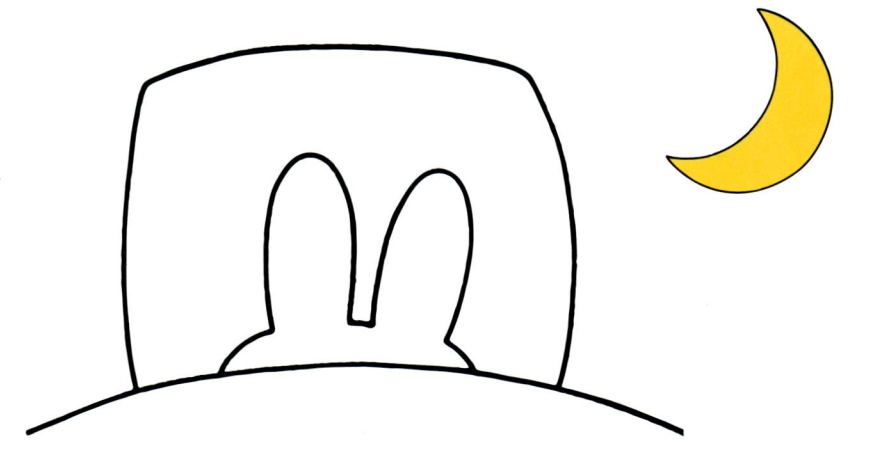

....

Moved to a cot

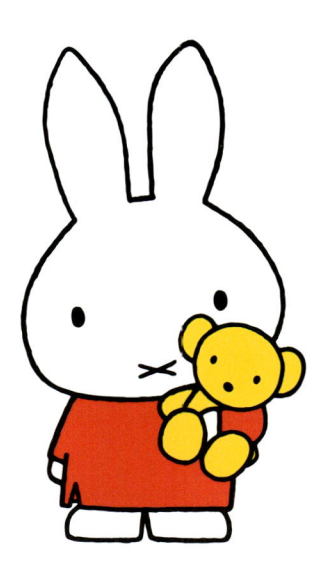

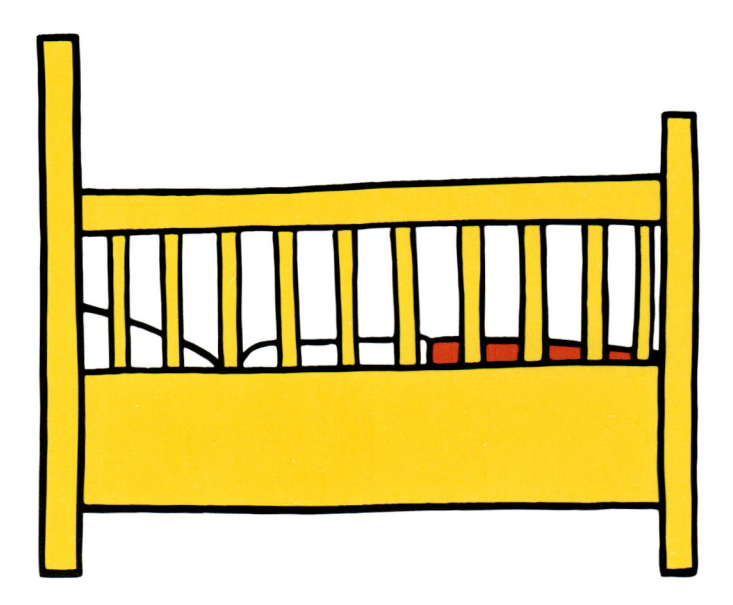

....

....

Favourite bedtime stories

....

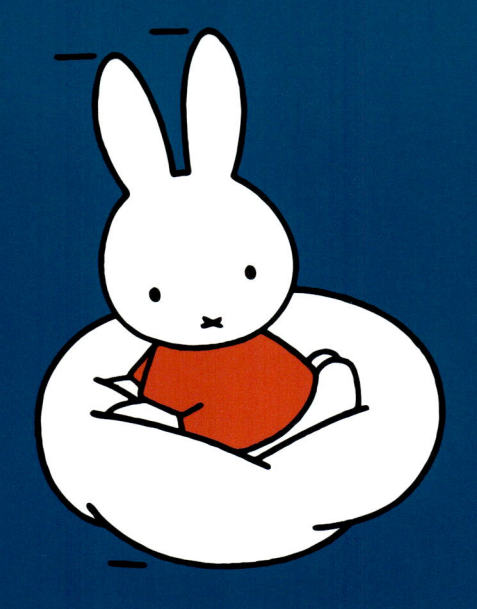

Favourite lullabies

....

Photograph

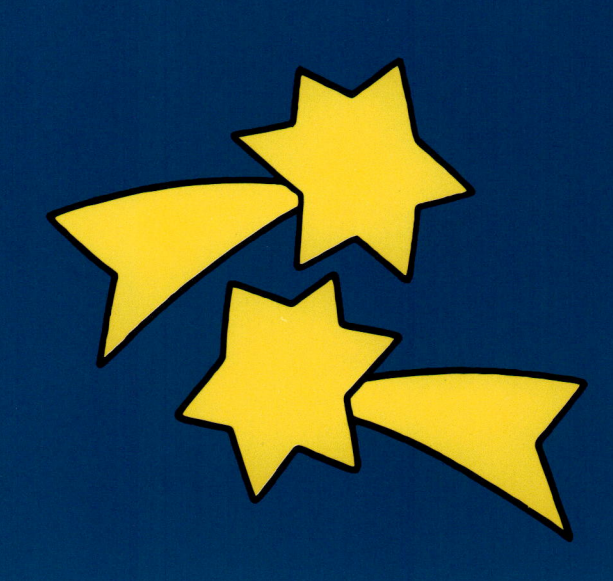

Baby's Meals

Weaned from the breast/bottle on ....

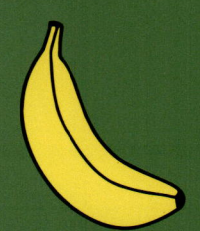

Date baby first: Ate pureed food ....

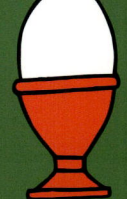

Ate solid food ....

Used fingers ....

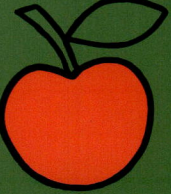

Held a spoon ....

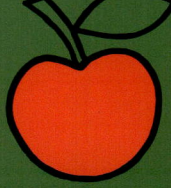

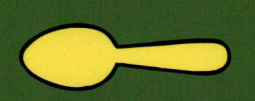

Sat in a high chair ....

Drank from a cup with help ....

Drank from a cup alone ....

Ate a complete meal ....

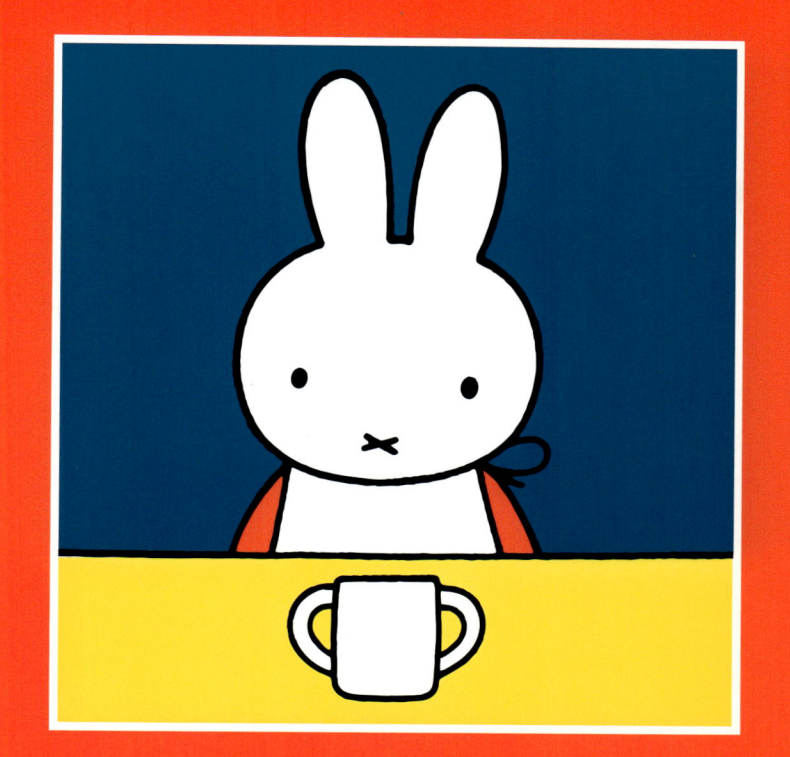

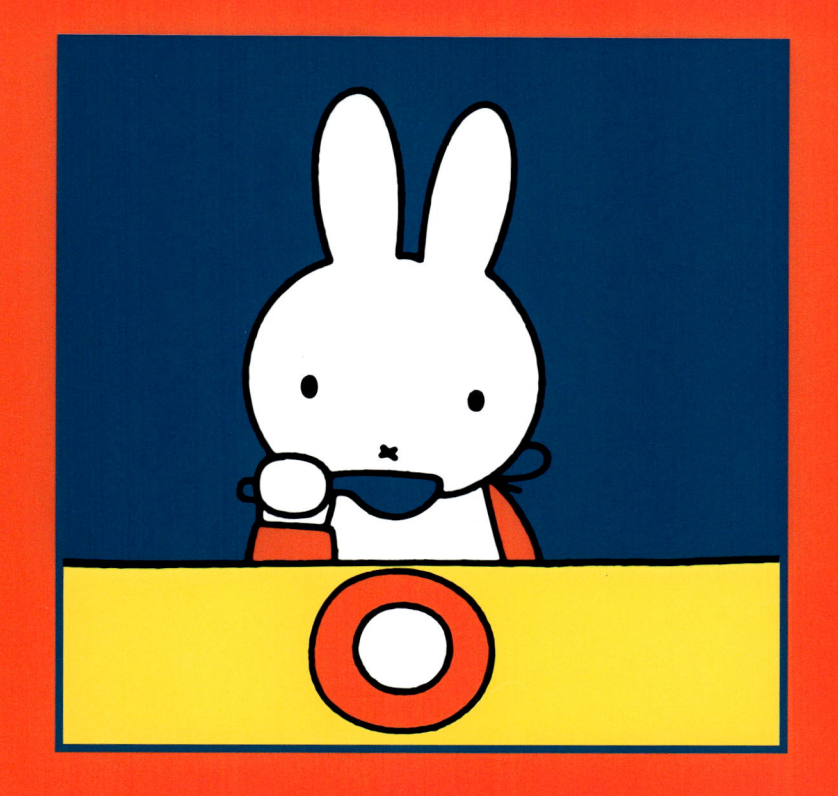

Food liked ....

Food disliked ....

Favourite food ....

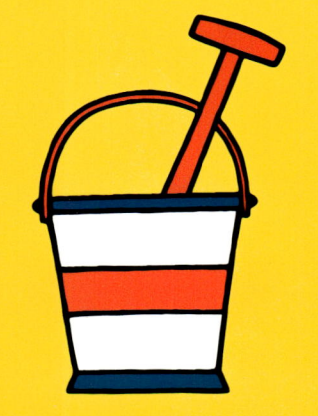

Best loved Toys

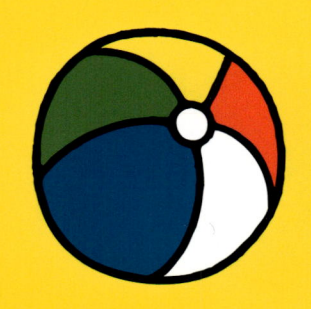

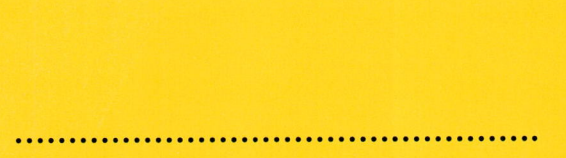

....

....

....

....

....

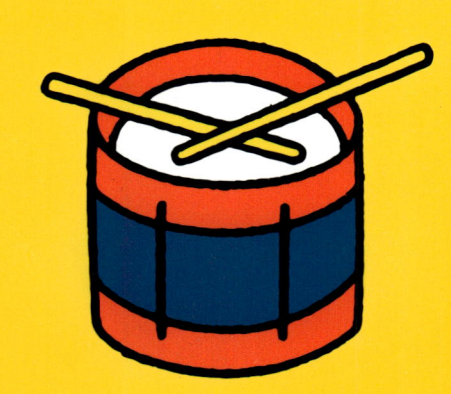

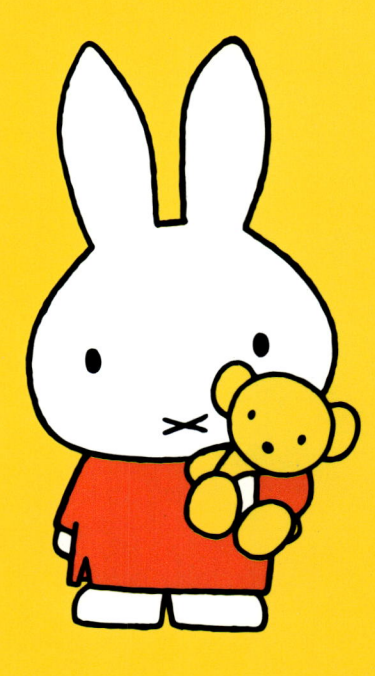

Favourite Things

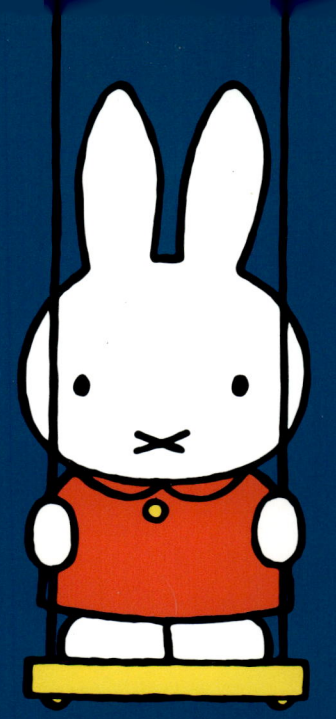

....

....

....

Photograph

Teething

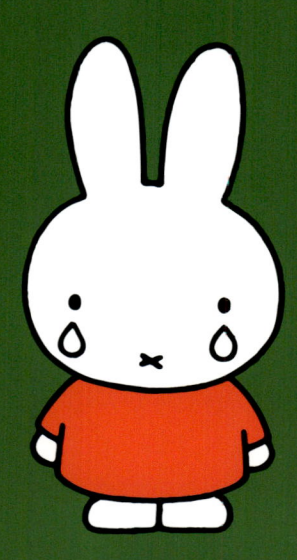

Favourite teething toy

....

First tooth appears

....

Photograph

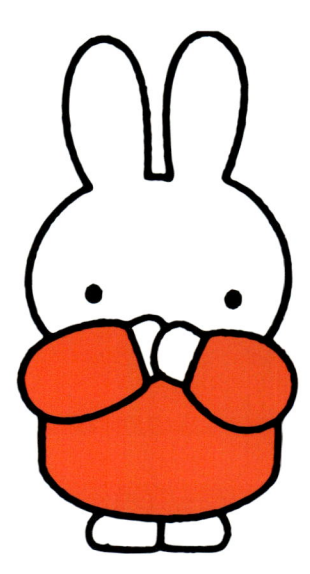

Growing Fast

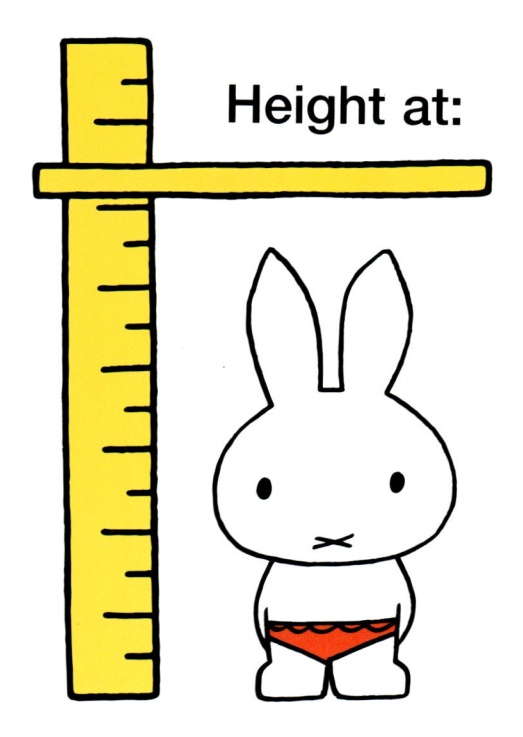

Height at:

1 year ....

9 months ....

6 months ....

3 months ....

1 month ....

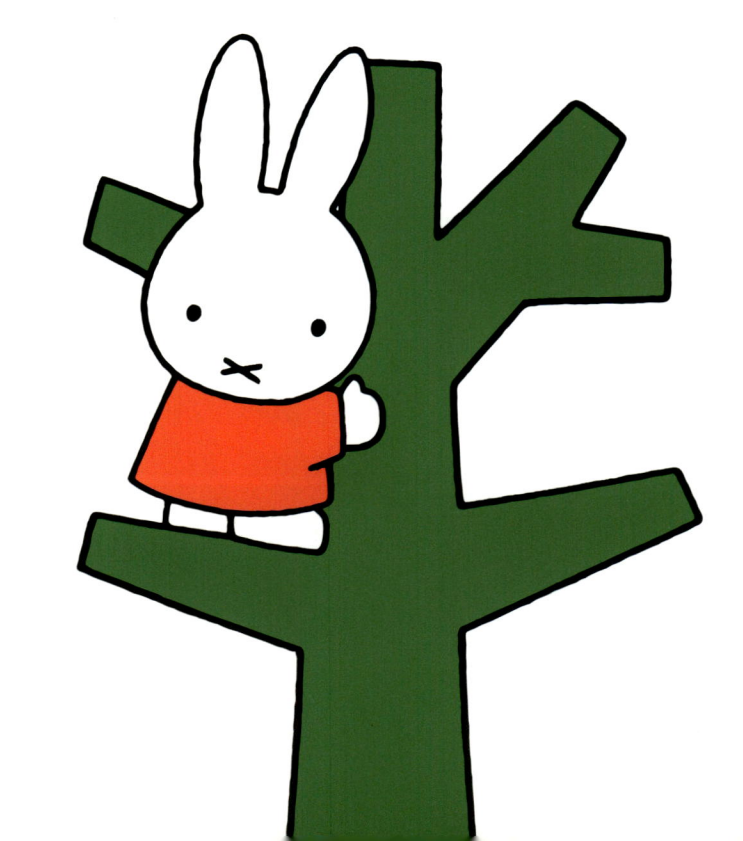

First Holiday

Where it was spent ....

Date of holiday ....

Length of stay ....

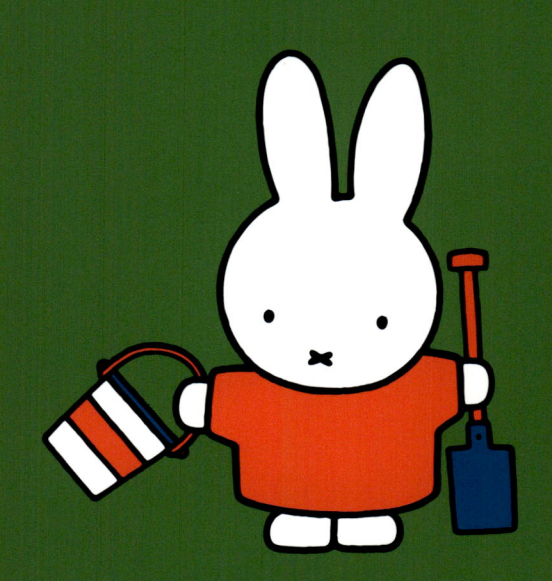

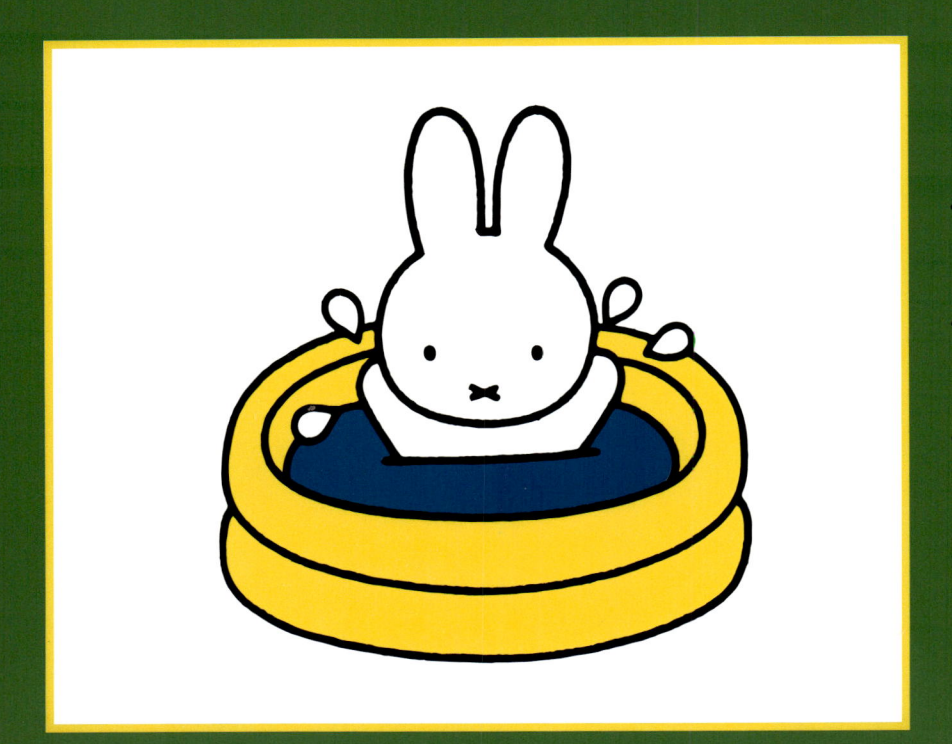

Memories to keep

....

....

....

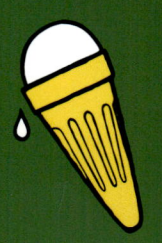

First Christmas

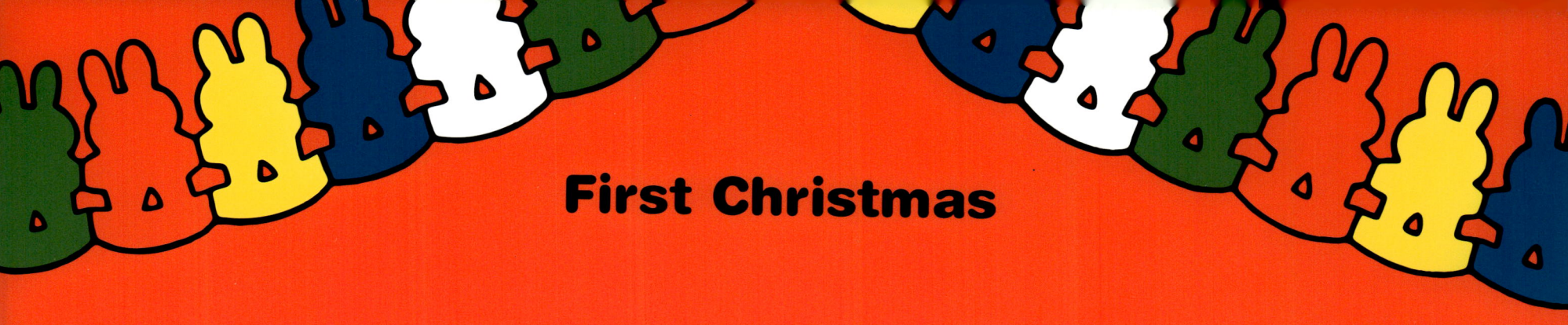

Favourite memories ....

....

Family and friends

....

....

....

Favourite gifts for Baby

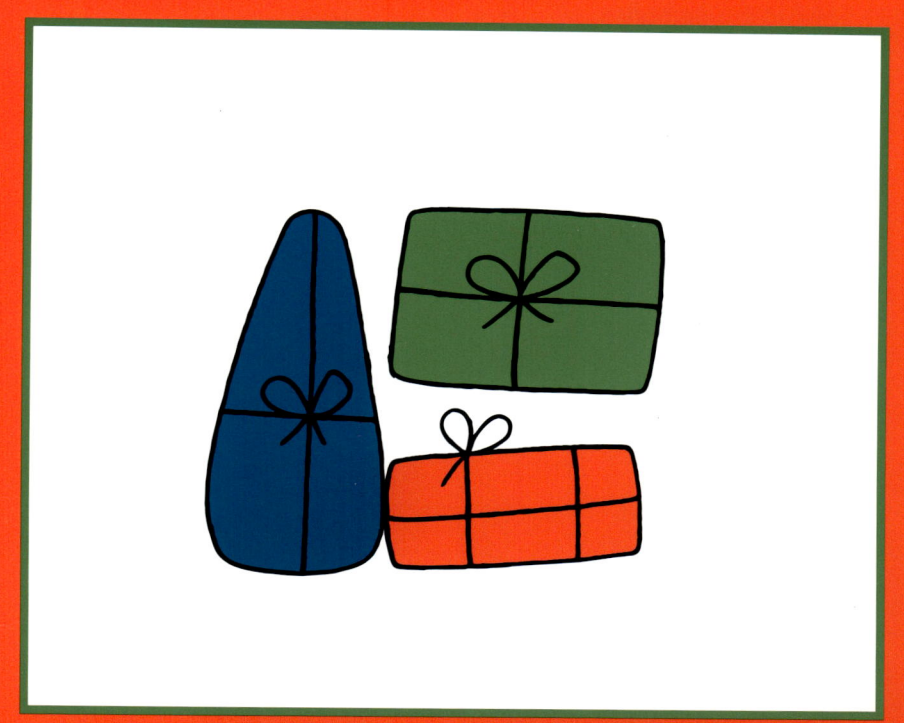

....

....

First Birthday

1

How it was celebrated ....

....

Who was there ....

....

Favourite memories ....

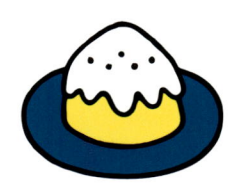

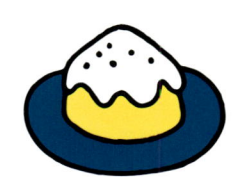

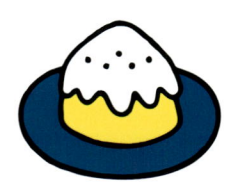

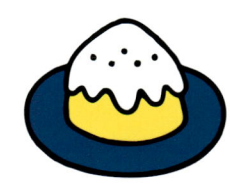

....

First Steps, First Words

When Baby first crawled ....

When Baby first walked ....

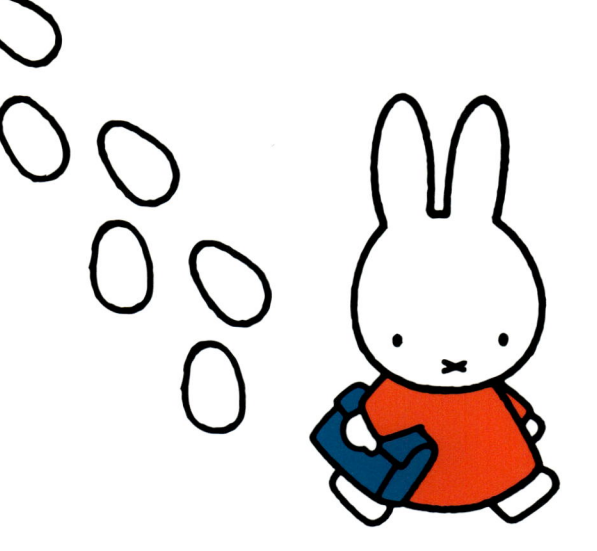

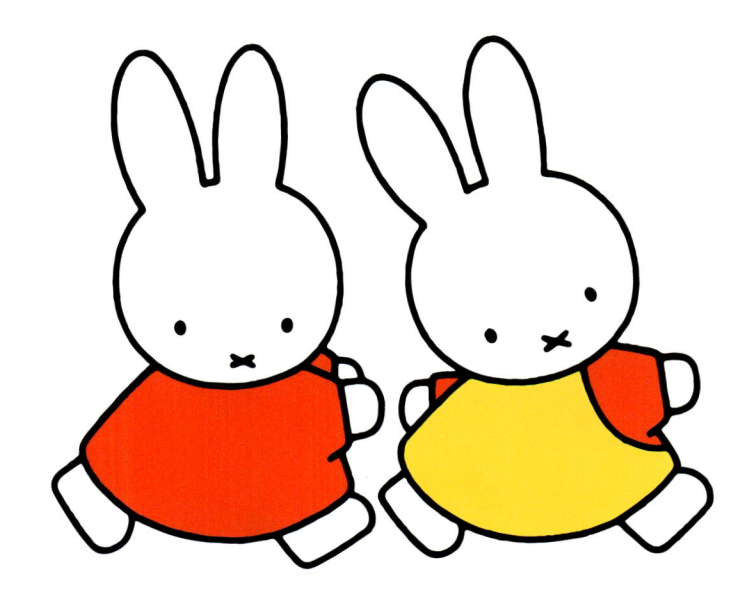

First word was ....

....

Next words were ....

....

First Events

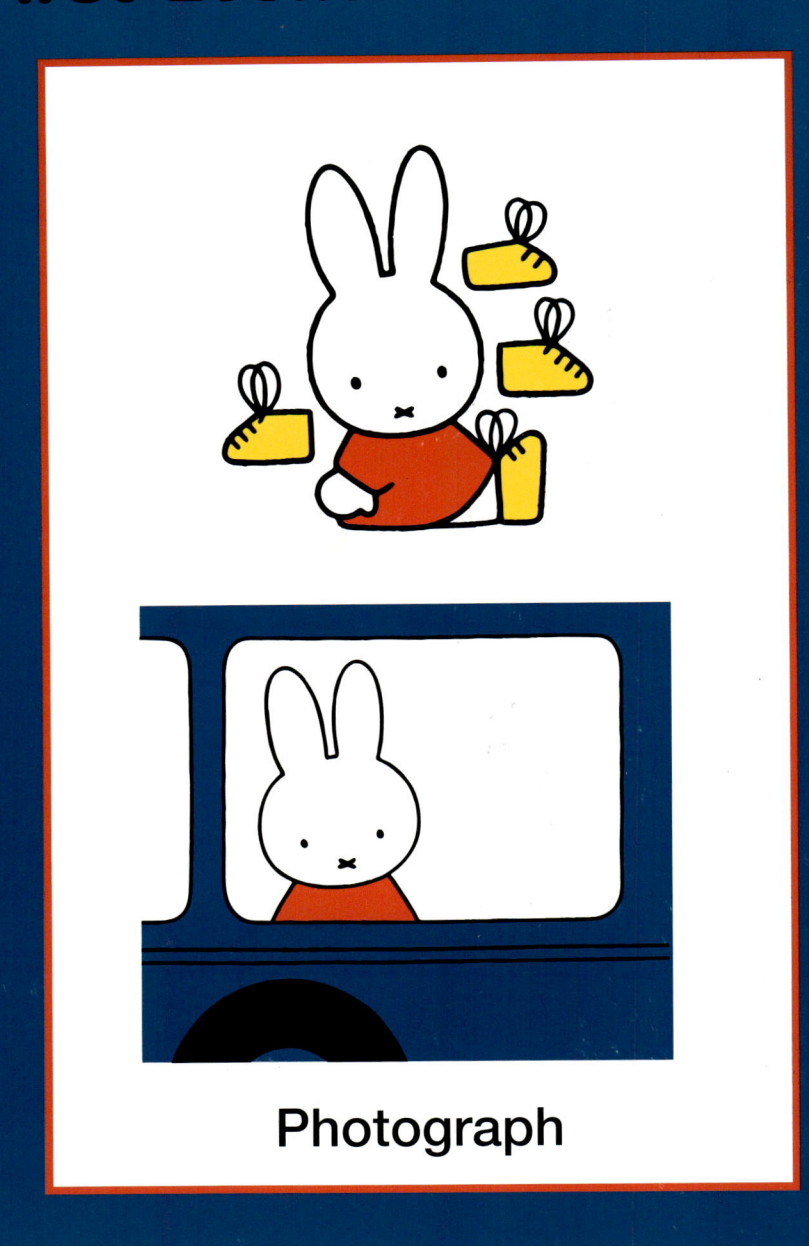

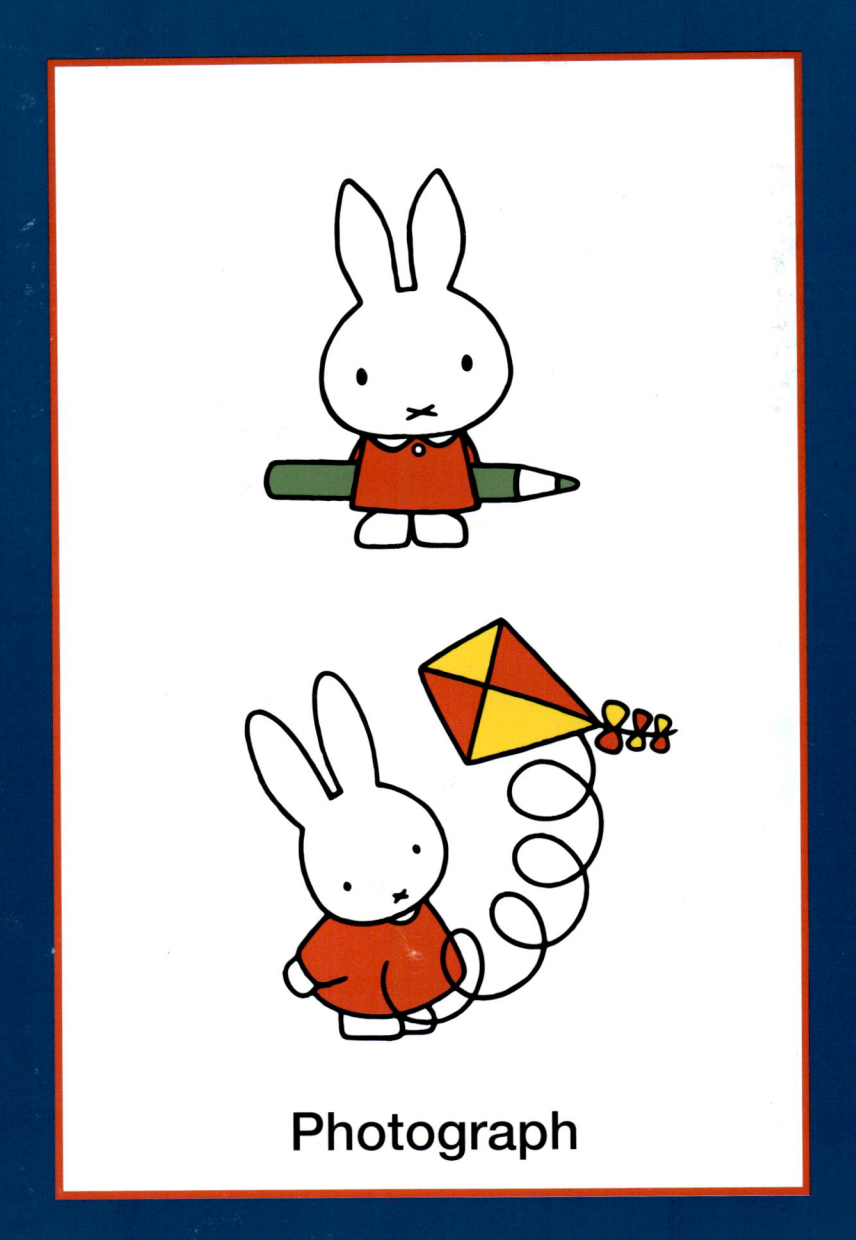

Photograph

Photograph